D1555693

# SLEEP AFTER MENOPAUSE

## Second edition

## Maria J. Sunseri, M.D. FAASM

Diplomate, ABSM, Subspecialty in Sleep Medicine

American Board of Sleep Medicine

American Board of Psychiatry and Neurology (ABPN)

ABPN, Subspecialty of Clinical Neurophysiology

American Board of Clinical Neurophysiology

With a bonus chapter on Sex After Menopause by Marcia Klein-Patel, MD PhD

Chief of the Women's Institute of Allegheny Health Network

Dedicated to all women…
and the people who love them.

Sleep After Menopause, 2nd Edition
ISBN: 9781076681362

Book objective/disclaimer: This book is intended to empower women with the information and education of how our bodies work and how to keep them healthy. It is not intended to replace individual doctor-patient relationships or the advice that those relationships confer. My hope is that this knowledge will give women the tools that they need to start the dialogue with the right health care professional, and alert them to the fact that they need further medical evaluation if that is the case.

# TABLE OF CONTENTS

# INTRODUCTION

*"I am starting to go through the changes of menopause and my friends say that I'll never sleep again... What am I going to do?"*

Does this sound familiar? If so, you are not alone. I have heard it many times.

I am a board-certified sleep medicine specialist, neurologist, and clinical neurophysiologist. I am also a postmenopausal woman. I sleep well, not perfectly, but quite well. I speak to you about the latest scientific knowledge, and with experience and insight to give you the tools to traverse this bridge in your life with some guidance and purposeful methods to counteract the whirlwind of negativity in which many women find themselves at this juncture in their life.

Women passing through menopause are not necessarily in a pathological state, although our bodies may feel out of control at times. Menopause is a natural passage. To make this journey less chaotic, we need to pay attention to our bodies as they change, so that this can be empowering rather than debilitating. Some women do have symptoms that require medical attention. Others just need direction that I hope you will be able to gather from this book. And if you need more help beyond what you learn here, do not be shy about getting that help. First, I will present what we understand to be normal about sleep and what are some issues that raise concern, to help you differentiate with your doctor what can be addressed naturally and what should be investigated further with medical testing such as a sleep study (polysomnogram), laboratory (blood) studies, or a consultation with a sleep specialist. Some women may need medication because their symptoms are severe, but most women just need to know how their bodies function, what is changing, and how to optimize their sleeping situation. Every woman does not need a pill.

I want to empower you with the knowledge of how your body sleeps: that is, your circadian rhythm, which is your internal clock, changes to your body temperature, and attention and awareness of your surroundings. I want to help you avoid letting goofy thoughts parade in your head that raise your anxiety and convince you that there is something so **wrong with your brain** that you will **never** sleep again. I cannot tell you how many patients come in feeling this way. This is one of the biggest factors that **perpetuate** a person's insomnia.

of REM sleep, but we know that it is essential for life. Mouse studies where the rodents were deprived of REM sleep demonstrated that they got sick and eventually died. We are essentially hallucinating when we dream, exciting neurons in our brain that conjure up disjointed images and melt them together, sometimes making very silly stories. Some research suggests that this is the time when our brains are sorting through the experiences, visual and other sensory input that happened throughout our day, trying to make sense of it, laying down memory in the temporal part of our brain, in our hippocampus (7). This may be like "defragging" our brains, similar to defragging a computer or "spring cleaning" a closet. Anyone who has ever let their spring-cleaning go undone knows the disastrous consequence if this is not done for a long time. The amount of time that we normally spend in REM sleep each night is around 20-25% of our total sleep time. This remains constant throughout all of our adult life. In NonREM sleep there may be some dreaming, but it is not so elaborate, and we are not in that unique physiologic state of being paralyzed. In NonREM sleep, stages N1 and N2 are sometimes referred to as "light sleep" and you can be easily awakened from these states of sleep. This sleep is not necessarily very refreshing but can take up to 60% of our total sleep time. Stage N3 sleep, on the other hand, is what is called "deep sleep" or "Slow Wave Sleep" (SWS). This is the deep sleep that is prominent in the first third of the night, from a circadian rhythm point of view. It is linked to our body temperature and hormone production. Many people are missing much of this deep sleep stage because of late night schedules. It is the "deep sleep" that children are typically in when they fall asleep on the ride home when the family is out past their bedtime and they are impossible to awaken and are often confused. The majority of SWS occurs in the first third of the night. Growth hormone production peaks at this time. It is the state of sleep where many other beneficial effects occur for our immune system. It is thought that we lose some SWS as we age, but there is disagreement about this in the sleep field.

## Normal sleep stages

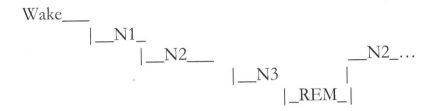

When we lie down to go to sleep, we are not conscious of the moment that we fall asleep. Studies show that we have amnesia for about five minutes of time before sleep onset (8). That is why we do not remember the exact time we fall asleep.

Have you ever watched someone fall asleep? It is an amazing process to watch. First their eyelids get heavy and they blink slower. If they are sitting, their head will tilt or drop because their neck muscles are relaxing.

Electrophysiologically, what we can see when someone is falling asleep is that their eyes start rolling, their muscle tone relaxes, and their brain waves slow down. Then, in N1 sleep we see sharp waves appear in the middle of the brain, called Vertex Sharp Waves of Sleep. In N2 we see these Vertex Sharp Waves but also short runs of fast waves hanging on to the end of the Vertex Wave making what is called a K-Complex. These K-Complexes emanate from structures deep on either side of the brain called the Thalamus. The Thalamus sits above our Hypothalamus (HT) which controls our sleep and wake switch, our internal "clock", and our body temperature. The HT is sometimes referred to as our "thermostat".

Next, we drop into N3 sleep which is that deep slow wave sleep (SWS). This is the sleep that is so deep that you just do not want to wake from when you have fallen asleep on the couch and someone wakes you to go up to bed. You may wake and be quite disoriented. In this stage, we have high voltage, very slow brain waves.

An important physiologic aspect of sleep is how closely it is linked to our body temperature rhythm. As we will discuss later when reviewing circadian rhythms; almost all our cells in our body have clock genes that help our cells tightly link our body temperature, hormones and sleep to our circadian rhythm. Our circadian rhythm is linked to our "light-dark" cycle. We fall asleep based on a few factors being present. This is one of the most important parts of successfully maneuvering though a phase in life that is disrupting your sleep such as menopause, high anxiety, or high stress. You must optimize every other factor influencing your sleep that you can! But to do this you need to understand how things work... So, here's the deal. We fall asleep as our body temperature drops. (9) This is extremely important, so I am going to say it again. ***We fall asleep as our body temperature drops.*** This is the reason many people can remember having difficulty falling asleep as a child on a hot summer night if they did not have air conditioning. This is also why it is so important not to exercise close to bedtime, because the exercise will increase your core body temperature making it difficult to fall asleep. Even the slightest increase in body temperature can disrupt our sleep and wake us.

When we are perimenopausal or postmenopausal and having hot flashes, a woman's core body temperature is raised just a fraction of a degree, but that is enough to disturb her sleep and wake her. Even hormonal changes that affect our body temperature right before or during our menstrual period can cause sleep to be disrupted. Many women have noticed that their sleep is disturbed just before or during their menstrual period. This can even cause a problem for young girls who are just starting to menstruate. This is often due to their bodies being just a little warmer at this particular time in their cycle. In the perimenopausal time period, this appears to be augmented. Having said this, it may seem surprising that there is research that showed that warming the feet with a warm foot bath in the evening tends deepen SWS (10). You may notice this when going in a hot tub too, but it may take longer to cool off. This is because your body is facilitating heat loss through your skin, helping to facilitate core body temperature loss. This may take some time, anywhere from 25 minutes to 100 minutes so do not expect to fall asleep right afterwards. This is called "*thermal inertia*". We will talk more about this later.

Sound disrupts sleep too. I often remind my patients that you are unconscious when you are asleep, but you are not deaf! This is the reason that falling asleep with the TV, music, or even certain sound machines in the background, is not a good idea because every change in the sound of the tones may cause a micro-arousal in the brain's sleep, disrupting it. This may fragment your sleep, repeatedly arousing you from deep stage N3 SWS or REM sleep to the light sleep of N1 and N2. That is why I suggest a continuous sound, like a basic floor fan or window fan. A ceiling fan does not make a loud enough sound or monotonous enough sound and sometimes has a clicking intermittent sound. The floor fan provides both cooling and a monotonous sound to drowned out any intermittent sounds that will cause any brain arousal or disturbances.

It is important to remember that we do not know the exact moment that we fall asleep. We all arouse or wake multiple times through the night, but we roll over, maybe adjust our pillows, and fall back to sleep and never remember waking when we get up in the morning. However, if we "alert" ourselves each time we wake, looking at the clock and making note of the time, or pressing the light on our smart phone to check the time, we will actually **produce** and **perpetuate** insomnia and even cause something called Sleep State Misperception without even knowing that we are doing it. What happens is that when we are super-conscious of waking and we fall back asleep we do not feel like we are sleeping. We have amnesia for the actual time of falling asleep, but then we wake and "alert" ourselves over and over with the passing of the clock time such that we do not feel that we have slept in the intervening time even though we did sleep. This is the premise for why we ask people to get out of bed if they are not sleeping, to avoid this misperception.

Women and men spend a lot of money on sleep aids. Most sleep aid medications last just 3-4 hours and increase stage N1 and N2, light sleep. They do not enhance stage N3 (SWS) which is the deep restorative sleep that we want, and they may actually decrease it. REM sleep is suppressed by some antidepressants, even though it may seem like you are dreaming more. It is just more vivid dreaming. There is strong internal pressure for REM sleep to stay consistent throughout our lifespan unless there is something interfering with it like sleep apnea, where the person has obstructed breathing in REM sleep.

***So how much sleep do we need?*** There are lots of articles telling us how much sleep we need, and I just said a few paragraphs ago that REM sleep is essential for life. The National Sleep Foundation (NSF) recommends 7-9 hours of sleep each night. (11) This is not a mandate for 7-9 hours of sleep per night, but rather support for general sleep needs that are constantly being sacrificed in our 24/7 world of expectations.

There is more and more evidence supporting the importance of sleep for the immune system, metabolism, the effects on insulin resistance and even cellular aging. And so, thoughts appear like *"Oh no, just now when I am going through menopause, gaining weight, I have the world on my shoulders, and I'm not sleeping!"* There is no absolute number that is perfect for everyone, but most people need between 7-9 hours of sleep. The key is that you get sufficient sleep so that your body feels rested. *Take note of how you sleep when on a relaxing vacation or a quiet weekend.* This will give you an idea of how much sleep you need. Think of the time in your life when you slept best. What were the circumstances? What was the timing? Were you a night owl or more of a morning person? How much did you sleep then?

M. J. Sunseri, M.D.

# VIEW (1) OF ADULT HUMAN BRAIN

**T=THALAMUS**
**HT= HYPOTHALAMUS**

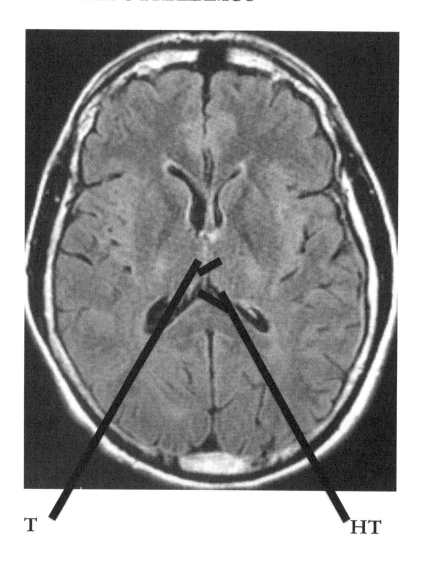

T                                          HT

# CIRCADIAN RHYTHMS

*Pam (not her real name) travels back and forth to Europe to see family every Christmas holiday. She has a week off and loves travelling. She has been doing this for many years, but she does not seem to be able to adjust as easily as she used to adjust. Her whole body seems to be out of sync for weeks after returning home.*

We all have a circadian rhythm. This is our internal rhythm, our body clock, that is linked to different parts of our day. This guides when we naturally fall asleep and wake, when we are hungry, our internal body temperature fluctuations, and many metabolic and hormonal processes. This cycle is typically a little longer than 24 hours, closer to 25 hours. Our eyes are the conduit through which we synchronize to the light and the dark to help to align our circadian rhythm to the world's 24-hour day. Light goes through our eyes and suppresses the secretion of melatonin from the pineal gland. This is a gland that sits in the middle of our brain. When it gets dark, melatonin is secreted, and this helps us to become sleepy in the evening. However, many other cells and organs in our body are also involved in this circadian process. Even our intestines have a "clock". The time that we eat influences our circadian rhythm and vice versa. We use this feature to help people who are travelling to another time zone minimize their "jet-lag" by shifting their meals and their light exposure towards their destination time zone before they leave. Did you ever notice that when you travel to other time zones and if you feel the effects of "jet lag", you don't feel hungry when meals are served and you are famished at other times? Or sometimes you even feel nauseated? That is because your digestive system is still on your "home" time-zone circadian rhythm.

The same happens with our temperature rhythm and this really confuses our sleep rhythm. You see, we fall asleep when our body temperature drops, and we stay asleep as long as our temperature stays low but when it starts to rise again, we wake up. We can fall asleep at other times if we are tired enough, but we will probably not stay asleep because of our temperature regulation being out of sync with the light-dark cycle of our destination. This is an important aspect of normal sleep that is affected with perimenopause and menopause. Although you are not "jet-lagged" in menopause, situations occur such as commitments to work and family life, as well as trying to make up for disrupted sleep, which necessitate understanding your personal circadian rhythm in order to maximize your success in making changes to maneuver these challenges.

Most women have understood that "hot flashes" can wake them up and disrupt their sleep but they do not know **why** and therefore they do not know how to adjust their life and their sleeping environment to minimize this. Every woman does not need a pill. Some women may need medication because their symptoms are severe, but most women just need to know how their bodies function, what is changing, and how to optimize their situation so they can sleep. This in turn will avoid the superimposed sleep disorders that follow and turn into chronic insomnia.

It was once thought that we had one "clock" and that was in our suprachiasmatic nucleus (SCN) in the brain which controlled everything. The SCN is a part of the hypothalamus that we talked about before, (VIEW 1) in the center of our brain. However, now we know that most cells in our bodies have a clock rhythm that can be influenced by our environment. The most powerful influence on this rhythm is *light*. That is why we use light to "shift" and to stabilize our sleep-wake rhythms. It is also one of the reasons there is so much confusion today regarding sleep. Over the last 100 years artificial light has dramatically altered our world. There are so many positive inventions that make life easier, but we need to recognize when we must be in control of our technology so that it does not inadvertently cause us harm. This is what I mean by understanding our bodies and how they function so that we can adjust when our body changes, to optimize our sleep. For instance, this is the reason that I will later propose *avoiding light in the evening, dimming the computer light in the evening, and stopping it all together at least 2 hours before bedtime*. This includes the light from our smart phones, so look for and turn on the "night light" setting on your phone and other devices.

In the two-process model of sleep regulation (12) there is the homeostatic system (**S**) that accumulates "sleep debt" starting when we get up in the morning, until we go to sleep at night. The other system is our circadian system (**C**) which is comprised of our inner clock and the timing of certain hormone production such as cortisol and growth hormone as well as body temperature. When these two systems, Process **S** and Process **C** are aligned, then our circadian system helps us to stay awake as we go through our day even though we are accumulating more and more "sleep debt". Once we get to a certain point however, after melatonin is secreted with the dimming of the light "zeitgeber" or "trigger", and our body temperature starts dropping, our circadian system then switches to promote sleep and the two systems are then ready for sleep. This means that with these two systems aligned, our bodies are in an ideal state for sleep. As we sleep, our homeostatic system (Process **S**) is "paying off" our sleep debt so there is very little reason for us to stay asleep except that the circadian system (Process **C**) is still in strong sleep promoting mode. Once our circadian system (Process **C**) is ready to wake, we wake for the day... if these two systems are in alignment.

If these Processes are out of alignment such as with "jet lag", shift work or a Delayed Sleep Phase where a person's internal rhythm/circadian rhythm is delayed several hours, i.e. a real "night owl", then we have problems…but these are fixable problems. We can change our behavior, change our light exposure, and if needed, use some melatonin to help get back on track.

If our system is disturbed because of abnormal temperatures, such as a hot summer night without air-conditioning, a fever, or more pertinent to this book's subject, perimenopausal or postmenopausal hot flashes, then methods to optimize our body temperature are most helpful.

# MENOPAUSE

Most of us can remember the ups and downs, and the trials and tribulations of puberty. Hormones were changing. Our bodies were changing. Some people knew what was happening to them and others did not. Well, menopause is a little like that, but the changes are occurring somewhat in the opposite direction.

So, with this background, let us talk about what is happening in the perimenopause and postmenopausal time period for us, mostly women of a certain age. To start, let's clarify the definition of menopause. Simply, **menopause** is defined as the last menstrual period. You are **postmenopausal** once you have gone one year without a menstrual period. Even though we are living longer, the average age of menopause has remained constant, around 51 years old, with a

M. J. Sunseri, M.D.

range of between 40-58 years old. Perimenopause is the time before and after menopause when a woman may be having some symptoms, but she is not yet postmenopausal.

A well-recognized issue at the time of menopause is that we tend to put on weight more easily and this weight is not distributed evenly but mostly around our middle body and our neck. This central fat raises our risk for health problems such as sleep apnea, diabetes, and high cholesterol and triglycerides. A small study out of Duke University suggests that women with type 2 diabetes going through menopause may have more sleep issues and more severe sleep symptoms during menopause than their peers without diabetes (13). There is an increased prevalence of thyroid problems for women at this juncture in life and that can upset our sleep, our energy, and our mood.

The change in our hormones is like going through the whirlwind of puberty all over again but in the opposite direction. However, a little bit of knowledge and a lot of laughter can get you through it! Learning to understand your body can help you roll with the punches.

Your estrogen will be decreasing and your FSH (follicle stimulating hormone) and LH (luteinizing hormone) are increasing. Estrogen receptors are ubiquitous (and I mean everywhere) throughout our bodies and therefore when estrogen levels change/decrease, this has influence in many body systems, including our brains.

There are several forms of estrogen but the following two are most effected; **estradiol (E2)** in part from the ovary and **estrone (E1)** which comes from fat tissue. E2 is reduced more than E1. Estrone sulfate (E1S) is the highest level of any estrogen and this drops from around 1000pg/ml in premenopausal women to an average of 350pg/ml in postmenopausal women. (14) There are a lot of estrogen receptors all over our bodies and in the brain, which influence blood flow, synaptic activity, and neuronal growth. When we are young, before perimenopause, we are bathed in estrogen! That is why our skin is soft and supple and our mind is quick. However, when our estrogen falls, this contributes not only to the cosmetic changes but also to the memory and cognitive symptoms that we notice in the perimenopausal time, and which sometimes causes distress.

My mother was a very smart and conscientious woman. Yet, I remember vividly her distress when she was going through perimenopause with no one to turn to and no knowledge of what was happening to her body. She became so upset with herself because she went through a STOP sign when driving during her perimenopausal period. She was so distraught at her mistake that she quit driving. She thought she had some awful disease that caused her to do such a careless thing. Later in life, when she realized she was ok, she began driving again.

Myself, I felt so lucky to understand what was going on. It still felt odd at times, but I got to have some fun with it. I would wake in the morning and tease my husband, asking him "who am I today?" because I felt so different from day to day. He would sing to me the John Mayer song "Your Body is a Wonderland" and we would laugh. Those of us who have traversed this bridge without trauma, have done so because of knowledge, preparedness, understanding and humor. That is what I hope to give to you.

Hot flashes are also a symptom of estrogen deficiency and occur when estrogen levels fluctuate widely. This may be why they are often so prominent right before your menstrual period in perimenopause. The first thing to understand is that it is **_not the level_** of your hormones **_but the SLOPE of the change_** in the hormone (i.e. how fast it is dropping) that makes you feel really symptomatic or out of control. (14) Don't panic, **_this will level out._** If you are lucky, your estrogen will drop in small steps like a staircase, instead of a roller-coaster.

So, do not be too alarmed with every symptom that you feel, but if it is really bothering you and **_persistent_**, then seek medical attention. So for instance, when you start to forget some little things that you never forgot before---you might wonder if this is this the beginning of Alzheimer's ... or is this just because your brain is used to a lot more estrogen than it is getting at the moment? Remember, those estrogen receptors are everywhere, including your brain, and they are used to being bathed in estrogen. Now they are having a kind of estrogen starvation. It may bother you today and perhaps tomorrow but is it still bothering you two weeks from now? Or did you return to your normal cognitive function? The same goes for your mood. If your mood is bad for a week and then back to normal, that is one thing but if it is bad for weeks on end and you cannot shake it, that is what I mean by persistent. Then it is important to seek medical evaluation for two reasons. The first reason is because some symptoms can be too overwhelming. We are all different and some of us may need to use hormone replacement therapy for a limited time to help **ease the SLOPE** of declining estrogen, weaning the woman slowly from one level of estrogen to another. The second reason is because every symptom is not due to menopause. Just because you may be perimenopausal does not mean that you are immune to having any other medical problem.

The next point I want to make is that temperature is extremely important when it comes to sleep. I know I have said this several times, but I cannot overstate it. Many women complain of being cold most of their life, and then they hit menopause and are accosted by hot flashes and night sweats and they may think that that is the extent of it. However, when it comes to sleep, *it just takes a fraction of a degree of temperature elevation to disrupt your sleep.* You cannot even measure it with a thermometer. But if you just touch your breastbone area, you will feel a warmth or perspiration even when the rest of your body is cool or even cold! Your body is trying to dissipate the rise of heat by an increase in peripheral temperature in your hands and feet, a decrease in skin resistance associated with sweating, and then a reduction in your core body temperature. So, you see, your body is trying to help regulate your body temperature, trying to cool you down by sweating, to dissipate that heat. You need to help by doing things to cool your body down. Knowing this, try not to get too upset, angry and frustrated when you wake: this may only serve to heat you up!

A lesser known fact is that the perimenopausal changes can start to occur even 10 years before a woman goes through menopause. (14, 15) If you do not know what is happening, then you are much more likely to become anxious about "unexplained" sleep disruption and adopt sleep behaviors that are counterproductive. If you understand what is happening, it may still be aggravating when you have a disrupted night's sleep for a few days in a row, but you know that you can turn it around with some basic tools that will be reviewed in detail with the modified behavioral portion of cognitive behavioral therapy for insomnia (CBT-I). Please do not just skip ahead to that chapter yet☺. My aim is to be brief, but I want you to understand the "cognitive" part first, so you know **why** you are doing certain things and understand how your body sleeps naturally.

# THE PERFECT STORM

The average age for menopause is still around 51 years old. At 50, most of us have a lot on our minds, with family issues, health problems and the death of loved ones, financial issues, job stressors and children. We are often carrying the major responsibility for family concerns as the younger generation is just starting out, and many of us are taking care of parents as well. Our bodies are changing, and not necessarily in a positive direction. Even if we are very diligent about our diet and exercise, we cannot reverse the inevitable effects of aging that start to show, despite our best efforts. So, when you wake in the night with a hot flash or for another reason, it is easy to get pulled into a line of negative thinking and worrying about all the different things we have on our minds. But trying to resolve these problems when we are sleep deprived and frustrated because we are not sleeping is futile. We all know this. Data from the National Health Interview Survey, 2015 (16) reported that perimenopausal women are more likely to sleep less than 7 hours on average: postmenopausal women were more likely to have trouble falling asleep and staying asleep: and postmenopausal women were more likely to wake not feeling rested. Thus, the total time of sleep was more effected in the perimenopausal woman whereas the quality of the sleep was more effected in the postmenopausal woman.

So, how does this happen to so many otherwise healthy women? Well, we just reviewed in the previous chapter how our estrogen levels are dropping in the perimenopausal period and how this effects our brain and our temperature regulation in sleep. Hot flashes are the bodies' way of trying to help us cool off but that takes time and that time… that ***thermal inertia***, takes away time from our sleep. We know that we need to keep our core body temperature cool to maintain sleep. So, the perimenopausal woman is going to get less sleep due to this temperature interruption. But we have tools to improve this!

What concerns me more is that postmenopausal

women are reporting more trouble falling asleep, staying asleep and poor-quality sleep. Their estrogen levels should be pretty low by now. The _**slope of any change**_ in hormone levels should not be causing any major sleep symptoms now. So, what is causing this worsening of their sleep quality? Is it just an extension of their perimenopausal sleep disruption? Or have they **perpetuated** the wrong habits and **"learned"** how not to sleep well?

A major life event such as a serious illness or death of a loved one, divorce or job loss, may in and of itself keep us up for a few days to weeks, and is an example of what was in the past called an "Adjustment Insomnia". However, the stress typically dissipates over time and this should be what is now referred to as a "Transient or Short-term Insomnia". So why do some of us continue to have trouble sleeping? It is not the _**stress**_ that **perpetuates** the trouble sleeping. That stress is now gone in most cases. Rather, it is the habits and thoughts that we adopt during this acute event, that makes this problem snowball into a major sleep disruption in our life.

So, let me elaborate on this a bit. The concept of Insomnia is built on the principle of the **3 P's**: namely, **Predisposing**, **Precipitating**, and **Perpetuating**. Predisposing may refer to our previous sleep habits being good or poor, our personality traits being anxious or relaxed. Precipitating is a factor that in this case essentially all women have, that is, the effects of perimenopause/menopause. However, this may also include other stressors which can occur at the same time or in tandem and be additive or even overwhelming. But it is the *Perpetuating* factors that cause the insomnia to continue and become **chronic**. I will say that again. It is the Perpetuating factors that cause the insomnia to become chronic. *These are the learned factors* and it is a *learned insomnia*. In the past, this was termed *psychophysiologic insomnia*. This is what contributes to postmenopausal women being more likely to have trouble falling asleep, staying asleep and not feeling rested. However, we have tools to improve this too!

There are certain stressors that may make you so upset such that you are not able to sleep well. For instance, when your child is sick, or you are going through a major financial stressor or divorce. You may have trouble falling asleep or find yourself waking through the night. You might even have a night where you do not sleep at all--- Be assured, _**you will sleep again**_! The body can go a week without food, but it cannot go without sleep. Your brain will fall asleep even in a dangerous situation such as driving because it needs sleep and it will take it. But those little catnaps do not make you feel refreshed. What you need to do is learn how to optimize your life for sleep in these situations----so when you're under stress and you are not sleeping well, you must be super diligent about the modified cognitive behavioral therapy (CBT-I) that you will learn in the coming chapters. We will also use sleep consolidation/restriction to jump start the process.   In a nutshell, you need to remember how your body sleeps (your circadian rhythm, attention to body temperature, attention to your surroundings,) and not let goofy thoughts parade in your head, raising your anxiety and convincing you that there is _something so wrong with your brain_ that you will _never_ sleep again. I cannot tell you how many patients come in feeling that way. This is one of the biggest factors that **_perpetuate_** a person's insomnia.

Next, with the frequency but unpredictability of hot flashes accept the fact that you **will** wake up when your body temperature rises, even just a little bit. So **when** you wake up, even if you do not feel hot, touch yourself in the vicinity of your neck and breastbone area and if you are warm or perspiring there... *it is the hot flash, your slightly elevated body temperature that woke you.* So do not let your anxiety start to rise..., throw off your covers, or stick your feet out to cool in the breeze of a fan ---a fast way to cool the core body temperature is through the feet--- or go get a cool cloth or gel pack from the refrigerator to put on your forehead and don't keep looking at the clock. I will propose later that you set your alarm and turn your clock around so that you do not even see your clock. Be confident, you know what woke you and when your temperature drops, you will fall back to sleep. Sometimes an aspirin can help and if you have been told to take an aspirin daily, take it at bedtime. Aspirin is sleep promoting, i.e. soporific. Melatonin also slightly decreases body temperature. You do not need to take a high dose; just 0.5 to 1 mg is enough. I did not take this nightly, but if I were waking warm frequently through the night (possibly during an estrogen hormone step-down) I would take some melatonin. If I have been exercising a lot and have aches and pains, I will take 1-2 aspirin at bedtime.

Some women have a major problem with hot flashes and can benefit from discussing with their gynecologist some natural remedies such as black cohosh. There are some medications that can be helpful, including gabapentin (Neurontin) (17) or some antidepressants like sertraline (Zoloft) and other selective serotonin reuptake inhibitors, SSRIs for short (18). Lastly, hormone therapy (HT) can be used, but there are risks that need to be weighed against the benefit that you are trying to achieve. Eventually you need to come off the HT and you will experience some of these symptoms anyhow when you come off them. However, it may be helpful, especially in those women in whom their estrogen is dropping precipitously (remember the **SLOPE of the change in estrogen level** is what matters). Then they can taper the dose more slowly to decrease symptoms that are out of control.

# WHAT TO DO?

First, I want you to ask yourself a few important questions to see if you need to see your medical doctor. There are some medical conditions that should be checked if you have any unusual (associated with shortness of breath), untimely (all night long), or otherwise odd night sweats (associated with other symptoms). As I mentioned before, the thyroid tends to cause problems at this time of life. This can be checked with a basic blood test (TSH, T4). Another simple blood test, a CBC with differential, can check for leukemia which can cause excessive night sweats. Some other testing can be done to look for other serious conditions (associated with some cancers and prolonged night sweats) if your medical history warrants it. Lastly, sleep apnea may cause night sweats, especially if it is severe. So, get a general physical exam and/or see your gynecologist if you have not recently. There are also a few sleep disorders that need medical attention if you have certain symptoms, so if you fall into any of these categories, PLEASE do not ignore these signs and symptoms. I have included a few simple questionnaires to help guide you. You need a few pieces of information to answer these questions.

A) your body mass index (BMI) from the table below

B) or you can calculate your BMI by taking your weight in kilograms (which is = your weight in pounds divided by 2.20462) divided by your height in meters squared (which is = your height in inches times 2.54 and divided by 100, which gives you your height in meters, then multiply the result by itself to give you your height in meters squared.)

C) measure your neck size in centimeters or inches

# M. J. Sunseri, M.D.

## Body Mass Index Table

| BMI | Normal | | | | | | Overweight | | | | Obese | | | | | | | | | Extreme Obesity | | | | | | | | | | | | | | | | |
|---|---|---|---|---|---|---|---|---|---|---|---|---|---|---|---|---|---|---|---|---|---|---|---|---|---|---|---|---|---|---|---|---|---|---|---|---|
| | 19 | 20 | 21 | 22 | 23 | 24 | 25 | 26 | 27 | 28 | 29 | 30 | 31 | 32 | 33 | 34 | 35 | 36 | 37 | 38 | 39 | 40 | 41 | 42 | 43 | 44 | 45 | 46 | 47 | 48 | 49 | 50 | 51 | 52 | 53 | 54 |

Height (inches) — Body Weight (pounds)

| Height | 19 | 20 | 21 | 22 | 23 | 24 | 25 | 26 | 27 | 28 | 29 | 30 | 31 | 32 | 33 | 34 | 35 | 36 | 37 | 38 | 39 | 40 | 41 | 42 | 43 | 44 | 45 | 46 | 47 | 48 | 49 | 50 | 51 | 52 | 53 | 54 |
|---|---|---|---|---|---|---|---|---|---|---|---|---|---|---|---|---|---|---|---|---|---|---|---|---|---|---|---|---|---|---|---|---|---|---|---|---|
| 58 | 91 | 96 | 100 | 105 | 110 | 115 | 119 | 124 | 129 | 134 | 138 | 143 | 148 | 153 | 158 | 162 | 167 | 172 | 177 | 181 | 186 | 191 | 196 | 201 | 205 | 210 | 215 | 220 | 224 | 229 | 234 | 239 | 244 | 248 | 253 | 258 |
| 59 | 94 | 99 | 104 | 109 | 114 | 119 | 124 | 128 | 133 | 138 | 143 | 148 | 153 | 158 | 163 | 168 | 173 | 178 | 183 | 188 | 193 | 198 | 203 | 208 | 212 | 217 | 222 | 227 | 232 | 237 | 242 | 247 | 252 | 257 | 262 | 267 |
| 60 | 97 | 102 | 107 | 112 | 118 | 123 | 128 | 133 | 138 | 143 | 148 | 153 | 158 | 163 | 168 | 174 | 179 | 184 | 189 | 194 | 199 | 204 | 209 | 215 | 220 | 225 | 230 | 235 | 240 | 245 | 250 | 255 | 261 | 266 | 271 | 276 |
| 61 | 100 | 106 | 111 | 116 | 122 | 127 | 132 | 137 | 143 | 148 | 153 | 158 | 164 | 169 | 174 | 180 | 185 | 190 | 195 | 201 | 206 | 211 | 217 | 222 | 227 | 232 | 238 | 243 | 248 | 254 | 259 | 264 | 269 | 275 | 280 | 285 |
| 62 | 104 | 109 | 115 | 120 | 126 | 131 | 136 | 142 | 147 | 153 | 158 | 164 | 169 | 175 | 180 | 186 | 191 | 196 | 202 | 207 | 213 | 218 | 224 | 229 | 235 | 240 | 246 | 251 | 256 | 262 | 267 | 273 | 278 | 284 | 289 | 295 |
| 63 | 107 | 113 | 118 | 124 | 130 | 135 | 141 | 146 | 152 | 158 | 163 | 169 | 175 | 180 | 186 | 191 | 197 | 203 | 208 | 214 | 220 | 225 | 231 | 237 | 242 | 248 | 254 | 259 | 265 | 270 | 278 | 282 | 287 | 293 | 299 | 304 |
| 64 | 110 | 116 | 122 | 128 | 134 | 140 | 145 | 151 | 157 | 163 | 169 | 174 | 180 | 186 | 192 | 197 | 204 | 209 | 215 | 221 | 227 | 232 | 238 | 244 | 250 | 256 | 262 | 267 | 273 | 279 | 285 | 291 | 296 | 302 | 308 | 314 |
| 65 | 114 | 120 | 126 | 132 | 138 | 144 | 150 | 156 | 162 | 168 | 174 | 180 | 186 | 192 | 198 | 204 | 210 | 216 | 222 | 228 | 234 | 240 | 246 | 252 | 258 | 264 | 270 | 276 | 282 | 288 | 294 | 300 | 306 | 312 | 318 | 324 |
| 66 | 118 | 124 | 130 | 136 | 142 | 148 | 155 | 161 | 167 | 173 | 179 | 186 | 192 | 198 | 204 | 210 | 216 | 223 | 229 | 235 | 241 | 247 | 253 | 260 | 266 | 272 | 278 | 284 | 291 | 297 | 303 | 309 | 315 | 322 | 328 | 334 |
| 67 | 121 | 127 | 134 | 140 | 146 | 153 | 159 | 166 | 172 | 178 | 185 | 191 | 198 | 204 | 211 | 217 | 223 | 230 | 236 | 242 | 249 | 255 | 261 | 268 | 274 | 280 | 287 | 293 | 299 | 306 | 312 | 319 | 325 | 331 | 338 | 344 |
| 68 | 125 | 131 | 138 | 144 | 151 | 158 | 164 | 171 | 177 | 184 | 190 | 197 | 203 | 210 | 216 | 223 | 230 | 236 | 243 | 249 | 256 | 262 | 269 | 276 | 282 | 289 | 295 | 302 | 308 | 315 | 322 | 328 | 335 | 341 | 348 | 354 |
| 69 | 128 | 135 | 142 | 149 | 155 | 162 | 169 | 176 | 182 | 189 | 196 | 203 | 209 | 216 | 223 | 230 | 236 | 243 | 250 | 257 | 263 | 270 | 277 | 284 | 291 | 297 | 304 | 311 | 318 | 324 | 331 | 338 | 345 | 351 | 358 | 365 |
| 70 | 132 | 139 | 146 | 153 | 160 | 167 | 174 | 181 | 188 | 195 | 202 | 209 | 216 | 222 | 229 | 236 | 243 | 250 | 257 | 264 | 271 | 278 | 285 | 292 | 299 | 306 | 313 | 320 | 327 | 334 | 341 | 348 | 355 | 362 | 369 | 376 |
| 71 | 136 | 143 | 150 | 157 | 165 | 172 | 179 | 186 | 193 | 200 | 208 | 215 | 222 | 229 | 236 | 243 | 250 | 257 | 265 | 272 | 279 | 286 | 293 | 301 | 308 | 315 | 322 | 329 | 338 | 343 | 351 | 358 | 365 | 372 | 379 | 386 |
| 72 | 140 | 147 | 154 | 162 | 169 | 177 | 184 | 191 | 199 | 206 | 213 | 221 | 228 | 235 | 242 | 250 | 258 | 265 | 272 | 279 | 287 | 294 | 302 | 309 | 316 | 324 | 331 | 338 | 346 | 353 | 361 | 368 | 375 | 383 | 390 | 397 |
| 73 | 144 | 151 | 159 | 166 | 174 | 182 | 189 | 197 | 204 | 212 | 219 | 227 | 235 | 242 | 250 | 257 | 265 | 272 | 280 | 288 | 295 | 302 | 310 | 318 | 325 | 333 | 340 | 348 | 355 | 363 | 371 | 378 | 386 | 393 | 401 | 408 |
| 74 | 148 | 155 | 163 | 171 | 179 | 186 | 194 | 202 | 210 | 218 | 225 | 233 | 241 | 249 | 256 | 264 | 272 | 280 | 287 | 295 | 303 | 311 | 319 | 326 | 334 | 342 | 350 | 358 | 365 | 373 | 381 | 389 | 396 | 404 | 412 | 420 |
| 75 | 152 | 160 | 168 | 176 | 184 | 192 | 200 | 208 | 216 | 224 | 232 | 240 | 248 | 256 | 264 | 272 | 279 | 287 | 295 | 303 | 311 | 319 | 327 | 335 | 343 | 351 | 359 | 367 | 375 | 383 | 391 | 399 | 407 | 415 | 423 | 431 |
| 76 | 156 | 164 | 172 | 180 | 189 | 197 | 205 | 213 | 221 | 230 | 238 | 246 | 254 | 263 | 271 | 279 | 287 | 295 | 304 | 312 | 320 | 328 | 336 | 344 | 353 | 361 | 369 | 377 | 385 | 394 | 402 | 410 | 418 | 426 | 435 | 443 |

# STOP-BANG QUESTIONNAIRE: (19)

1) Do you snore loudly? (louder than talking or loud enough to be heard through closed doors)
Yes_____          No_____
2) Do you often feel tired, fatigued, or sleepy during the daytime?
Yes_____          No_____
3) Has anyone observed you stop breathing during your sleep?
Yes_____          No_____
4) Do you have or are you being treated for high blood pressure?
Yes_____          No_____
5) Is your body mass index (BMI) greater than 35?  BMI= kg/m2   (table on pg. 46)
Yes_____          No_____
6) Age over 50 years old?
Yes_____          No_____
7) Neck circumference greater than 40cms or 16 inches?
Yes_____          No_____
8) Male gender?
Yes_____          No_____

If you answered **YES to 3 or more** questions above, you have a **high risk of obstructive sleep apnea (OSA)** and you should see your doctor for a sleep study to evaluate for this.

OSA is an especially important sleep disorder that can cause high blood pressure, early age strokes, early age heart attacks, memory loss, mood disorders, excessive daytime sleepiness as well as insomnia and more. It is treated simply by Continuous Positive Airway Pressure (CPAP) which is applied from a small device about the size of a bedside radio. This is attached to a tube with a mask that fits over one's nose. It delivers air pressure to stent the airway open so you can breathe on your own. It is just keeping your airway from collapsing. It is not a respirator. It is not sexy, but neither is snoring, and this will eliminate your snoring. For those who are frightened of it, I like to have them think of it as something from the classic futuristic cartoon, "The Jetsons".

There have been incredible advances with the technology of the CPAP machines. Most people do not have problems with the air pressure. The challenge lies in finding the right mask to make each individual person comfortable. There are many kinds of masks, so do not be shy…shop around. If you have difficulty breathing out or exhaling against the pressure, then a slightly different device, a BiPAP or bi-level positive airway pressure device can help. This provides a higher pressure when you inhale (inhalation) and a lower pressure when you exhale (exhalation).

If you are overweight, then losing weight will usually help improve OSA and in some cases can cure it, but you need to keep the weight off for this to be a viable solution.

CPAP is the gold standard, but if you do not tolerate this and your OSA is mild to moderate, then oral appliance therapy (OAT) may be an option for you. This is an oral device that fits over your teeth and uses your upper teeth (maxillary) to pull your lower teeth (mandibular) forward to open your airway in the back of your throat. This is especially beneficial in people who are not overweight but have OSA based on an anatomically small airway. In many cases, weight loss may still be helpful when combined with the oral appliance. The oral appliance therapy (OAT) that is worn at night brings the lower jaw forward and may be an alternative to CPAP or BiPAP.

Finally, upper airway surgery should only be done when there is a clear idea of what the problem is and what is going to be achieved by the surgery. Most adult surgeries will minimize snoring, but the patient may still have OSA and you should always have a sleep study done afterwards to assess the effectiveness of the surgery in curing the breathing abnormalities. The surgery that is most effective in curing OSA is the maxillomandibular advancement with genioglossus advancement surgery. This is where the lower jaw is broken and moved forward, and the tongue is moved forward. The degree of success of this surgery is dependent upon the surgeon and dependent upon keeping your weight under control afterwards as well. This type of surgery should be considered for patients with significant OSA who cannot tolerate CPAP therapy.

Inspire genioglossus stimulation is a newer therapy for selected patients who do not tolerate CPAP therapy. It is a pacemaker-like stimulation of the tongue that makes it protrude repeatedly to open the back of the airway.

Another pertinent sleep disorder whose symptoms should not be missed is Restless Leg/Limb Syndrome because this is a very treatable condition.

## RESTLESS LEGS (RLS) QUESTIONS:

1) Do you have an urge to move your legs that is accompanied by, or caused by, an uncomfortable and unpleasant leg sensation?
2) Do these symptoms primarily occur, or are they worse when you are resting or inactive, such as lying or sitting?
3) Are these symptoms partially or totally relieved by movement, such as walking or stretching, at least as long as you continue that movement?
4) Do these symptoms get worse or occur only in the evening or at night?

If these 4 components are present, then you may well have Restless Legs Syndrome (RLS) or the more proper term is Willis-Ekbom disease. However, since most lay people still refer to this as RLS, I will continue to as well. Many people have this occasionally, but if it is interfering with your sleep or your life you then may benefit from treatment and/or medication.

Most important however, is to evaluate for any underlying conditions that are predisposing to RLS such as untreated sleep apnea, pregnancy, renal failure, anemia, neuropathy, or iron deficiency. Any one of these conditions needs special attention if the RLS is to be treated effectively. Sometimes treatment of the underlying condition will make the RLS symptoms reduce to barely noticeable. We now understand that even if the patient is not anemic, the patients should have their blood counts and iron studies checked, including a ferritin level. If your ferritin level is low or low normal (less than or equal to 75) then you may benefit from treatment with supplemental iron, even if you are not anemic, until your ferritin is up to 75-100. This is thought to be due to the theory that despite normal iron in your blood, there may not be normal iron getting into your central nervous system, i.e. your brain and spinal cord. Iron is better absorbed if it is taken along with Vitamin C. Iron is usually taken as $FeSO4$, 325mg (or 65 mg of elemental iron) along with 100-200mg of Vitamin C daily, or up to three times a day if you can tolerate it without too much constipation. There is a liquid iron that claims not to cause so much constipation. It should not be taken by people with high iron stores (hemochromatosis) so please do not just take it without checking with your doctor first. Too much iron in the body can cause you a lot of neurologic and liver problems.

Although most RLS is idiopathic, which means it is from an unknown cause, it may also be necessary to check for things that contribute to neuropathy or nerve ending damage. This would include a hemoglobin A1C to check for diabetes, TSH for thyroid disorders, and B-12 level to check for nutritional deficiency, if indicated. There are also non-medicinal ways to improve RLS, including limiting caffeine, alcohol, and nicotine, all of which make RLS worse. Too much and too little exercise can bring on RLS.

The medications that help with RLS have undergone some changes in the recent years. Dopamine agonists have been used for many years for Parkinson's disease and first line for RLS in the past. However, they have come under much scrutiny because of their side effects causing compulsive behaviors such as gambling, hypersexuality and compulsive shopping (20) and problems with "augmentation" of the RLS, wherein they cause the symptoms of RLS to get worse and to start to occur earlier in the day. These include pramipexole (Mirapex), ropinirole (Requip), the skin patch rotigatine (Neupro) and levodopa/carbidopa (Sinemet) taken in small doses as a pill. Gabapentin (Neurontin) is an anti-seizure medication that has been effective but it has not undergone FDA approval for RLS, but its cousin drug, gabapentin enacarbil (Horizant), an alpha-2-delta ligand, which has an added compound to help with absorption, has received FDA approval for the treatment of RLS and is now a preferred first line therapy in certain cases.

About 33% of adults over the age of 30 will have RLS on occasion but that does not mean that it needs to be treated unless you are anemic, or your iron studies are abnormal.

The medications that treat the symptoms, do just that, only treat the symptoms, meaning that it only helps with the "disagreeable sensation" and it is not treating any underlying problem or curing anything. That is, unless you are being treated for one of the underlying disorders.

Medications that can make RLS worse include most antidepressants. Wellbutrin is the one antidepressant that does not worsen RLS.

The biggest mistake people make is confusing "nervous legs" or the habit of jiggling legs as restless legs. Even doctors make this mistake. RLS requires that the person have a disagreeable sensation that makes you feel like you *"have to move"* your legs. Once again, you need to have that disagreeable sensation that is **worse at night**, and **made better by movement**, to have a diagnosis of RLS.

Untreated OSA will make RLS worse until the OSA is treated. Anemia can make RLS quite severe until the anemia is treated. Sometimes RLS runs in families. In those cases, it typically starts to occur at a younger age. To reiterate, getting OSA treated will improve your RLS!

# COMMON PROBLEMS AND INSOMNIA DIAGNOSES:

The terminology for the classification of Insomnia has changed since I wrote the first edition of this book. Presently, insomnia is divided into Chronic Insomnia, Short-term Insomnia and Other Insomnia. The most common problem that I see with perimenopausal and postmenopausal women's sleep is a **Chronic Insomnia** that used to be called *Psychophysiologic Insomnia.* This is a fancy term for what is in essence "**learned insomnia**". Now I know that many of you who suffer with this are recoiling at the very thought that all you have suffered through could be something so simple.

However, when something occurs in life that causes a disruption of your sleep, a "Short-term Insomnia", it is easy to let things spiral out of control when everything you do seems to make things worse. That is because most people, and even many in the medical community, have not had enough knowledge about how our bodies sleep and **especially how this sleep changes at menopause**. After this goes on long enough, people *suffering with chronic insomnia* are *convinced* that there is something *wrong with their brain* so that they cannot sleep. They become anxious to even go to bed, because "they *know* they are not going to sleep". I am not in any way minimizing what you have been experiencing. I am simply stating that for people with Learned Insomnia there is a well-defined systematic way to recover and "***relearn***" how to sleep.

Many people have stressors that can cause a poor night's sleep. And most women will have some difficulty for at least some nights with their sleep when in the perimenopausal time period. The divergence between those who continue to have difficulties sleeping and those who go back to sleeping well is determined by what happens next. Good sleepers will typically say to themselves, "*Oh, I didn't sleep well at all last night. I am going to sleep like a log tonight!*" Others who have never had great sleep habits, or who are totally convinced by their friends and family that sleep is a problem at menopause from which they will never recover, will start to stress and become anxious, believing that something is wrong with their sleep or that they cannot sleep without a pill. They will say to themselves, "*Oh, I did not sleep at all last night; I am never going to sleep again*". Or they may say "*every postmenopausal woman*" in their family has a problem with sleep... the list of reasons goes on. But the body will sleep, as I said before. You can go a week without food, but you cannot go a week without sleep. Your body will sleep even in dangerous situations such as driving. You must quit getting in the way and learn to understand **how** your body sleeps and **when** your body sleeps so that you can optimize your chances of a good sleep.

Beth, (not her real name) is a classic example of patients who have come to see me wondering why they cannot sleep and thinking that *something is wrong with their brain.*

Her problem started about 5 years ago with some stress at work. At the same time, she was postmenopausal and noticed some hot flashes on and off, but not all the time. She had increasing administrative duties at work and would have problems sleeping, especially on Sunday nights. She eventually retired 3 years ago but her sleep problem became worse instead of better. She tried Ambien, a sleep aid, which worked at first but then quit working. She then tried other sleep medications; Sonata, then trazodone and then amitriptyline, on which she gained 25 pounds, so she quit taking it. Her sleep continued to get worse even though she went to bed every night at 11 PM. She did not fall into a good sleep until around 4 AM or 6 AM and then got up around 9 AM.

There are many examples of this type of *learned insomnia* in my practice, in both men and women. The *precipitating* factor or factors that initiate the trouble sleeping may vary but the *perpetuating* human nature that compels or tricks us into developing the psychophysiologic or learned insomnia is very similar from person to person. I want to teach you the cognitive and behavioral techniques to counteract these very natural human tendencies for incorporating the counterproductive thoughts and behaviors. We all have a bad night's sleep sometimes. *It is what we think about, what we expect, and what we do* with this "*bad night's sleep*", which **perpetuates** further bad sleep instead of good sleep.

So, in the case of Beth, the stress of her work is gone. She has retired. Her work stress was one of the main **precipitating** factors of her trouble sleeping initially. Why then is she still having trouble sleeping? In fact, she is having worse trouble sleeping! It is due to the **perpetuating factors**----that is, the **learned factors**. So, what did she do wrong? Let me start by saying that there is no fault here... it is just that she started down the wrong path because she did not have the knowledge about how her sleep works to help guide her differently.

We all have a poor night sleep occasionally, especially when we may be stressed. In Beth's case, she did not know that her hot flashes may be adding to her sleep disruption. She did not know to cool herself down for sleep and to use that knowledge to help get her back to sleep or recognize why she might be waking through the night. She initially had some restless night's sleep due to stress at work, made worse by hot flashes that disrupted her sleep. Then when she retired, she started spending way too much time in bed. Spending too much time in bed actually promotes insomnia! This brings up one of the most important points. It is extremely important to keep a *consistent wake-up time.* In fact, it is *most* important to get our sleep back on track. One's bedtime will eventually fall into place. Once you know your wake-up time, then you back out the average number of hours that you have been sleeping, and that should give you your bedtime.

In this example, if Beth had normally been a decent sleeper most of her life on a schedule of 11 PM to 6 AM and for the last few years she has only been sleeping 3-6 hours per night, then she should keep that wake up time of 6 AM. She should back out 6 hours and make a bedtime of 12 MN, for a total time in bed of 6 hours. *Once she is sleeping most of that time,* she can expand her time in bed by 15-minute increments if she is sleeping most of the time she is in bed. This does two things: it *consolidates* her sleep and it *reinforces* that she sleeps most of the time when she is in bed instead of being awake most of the time she is in bed. This improves her sleep efficiency!

Beth's sleep log before;

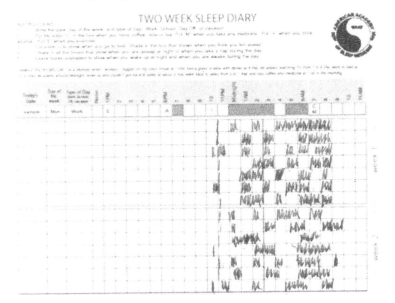

Then after realizing that;
1) Too much time in bed promotes insomnia so she must shrink her time in bed to just slightly more than the amount time she is actually sleeping, i.e. ~ 6 hours.
2) It is most important to keep a steady wake up time and bright light in the morning. So, she will get up at 6 AM and go to bed at 12 MN or later.

3) Understanding that you fall asleep as your body temperature drops and the optimal temperature for sleeping is 60-67 degrees, she adjusts the bedroom temperature.

Beth's sleep log after several weeks;

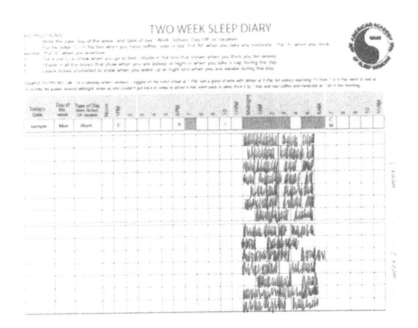

# CBT-I
# COGNITIVE BEHAVIORAL
# THERAPY FOR INSOMNIA
# MODIFIED AND WITH SLEEP
# CONSOLIDATION

So once the preceding medical disorders have been eliminated, the focus of evaluating and treating a perimenopausal and postmenopausal woman's sleep returns to identifying:

1)    When did your best sleep used to occur? What was your sleep schedule then? This will give you a clue to your natural circadian rhythm. Are you a night owl or a morning person? Does that coincide with the work/sleep schedule you are on now? What about your exercise schedule now?

2)    When did things start to go wrong: was it one event or a gradual accumulation of several events?

3)    What did you do to try to help yourself? Did it help? If it did not help you (like looking at the clock or taking sleeping pills), then **quit** doing it.

4)    Take some time to log your sleep for 2-4 weeks with the American Academy of Sleep Medicine (AASM) sleep logs on the following pages. Fill in the boxes when you think you slept.

## TWO WEEK SLEEP DIARY INSTRUCTIONS:

1. Write the date, day of the week, and type of day: Work, School, Day Off, or Vacation.

2. Put the letter "C" in the box when you have caffeine---coffee, cola or tea. Put "M" when you take any medicine. Put "A" when you drink alcohol. Put "E" when you exercise.

3. Put an arrow line (↓) down to show when you went to bed. Shade in the box that shows when you think you fell asleep.

4. Shade in all the boxes that show when you are asleep at night or when you take a nap during the day.

5. Leave boxes unshaded to show when you wake up at night and when you are awake during the day.

You will notice that each line starts at noon so that the night hours are in the middle of the page. This is so that you can better see consecutive night hours in bed, count them and see the consolidation over time as you proceed with the tools that I am giving you to use throughout this book.

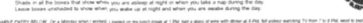

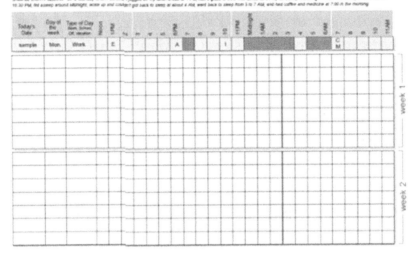

How to assess your sleep logs:

• First count how many boxes of sleep you filled in across each 24-hour period line across. (Partial boxes are added together). Take the average numbers of hours per night of the 14 days (add the number of hours from each night and then divide by 14 nights) and that is the amount of sleep on average you are getting. Keep this number handy because we are going to need this to consolidate your sleep, your *"sleep consolidator"*.

• Now look at what time you are waking for the morning (not just to go to the bathroom, but to get up for the day). Is this consistent from day to day? On the weekends or your days off, do you get up around the same time as during the week or do you sleep in many hours later? If you sleep in several hours later on your days off, then you may have a circadian rhythm problem----a Delayed Sleep Phase ----and you are essentially on "California time" (for East Coast women) and therefore your body rhythm is not ready to go to bed at 11 PM and get up at 7 AM. People like this want to go to bed much later and get up much later.

To the contrary, but less often, others are very early morning larks, an Advanced Sleep Phase---to an extreme degree and they fall asleep very early, around 8-9 PM and wake in the middle of the night, 3-4 AM, ready to start their day.

• Are you drinking alcohol, exercising, or eating close to bedtime? All these things will disrupt your sleep. Are you giving yourself any "down time" to wind down and relax?

• What is in your bedroom? Is there a TV?

Many people tell me that they cannot fall asleep unless the TV is on because they like the noise and silence makes them nervous. When you sleep, however, you are not deaf! You hear every change in intonation of people speaking on the TV or music notes changing up and down. This causes an arousal of your brainwaves and fragments your sleep. A better option is the monotonous sound of a floor or window fan. This drowns out the intermittent noises of cars passing by, the house "settling", people walking around, etc.... without a changing intonation that will arouse the brain. A ceiling fan typically does not make enough sound.

• Are there other things in your bedroom that remind you of things that may worry you? For instance, a desk with a pile of bills is not the thing you want to see right before laying down to go to sleep. Keep your bedroom free from as much clutter as possible. Let it be a stress-free environment for sleeping and sex... nothing else.

The concept of cognitive behavioral therapy has been used successfully in many areas of medicine, psychiatry, and psychology. The basic concept is to challenge and change misconceptions about a subject and combine this with behavioral changes. This method for use in insomnia has been supported with evidence-based medicine (21) for many years.

My impetus for writing this book was the fact that every woman eventually goes through menopause if she lives long enough. Some fly through without trouble and others do not, and they rarely have anyone knowledgeable about sleep to help them, so they really struggle. There are many other issues such as excessive bleeding and vaginal dryness that typically move to the top of the list, so their sleep suffers. They must use all their energy just to get from one day to the next, not knowing when or if their struggle will end. And the ones who have more than one problem, physical, social, or hormonal hit them all at once, often ending up in a tailspin. In my opinion, the medical system needs a comprehensive approach to the issues that a woman faces at menopause. In my approach, through education, I have successfully helped many women traverse this bridge in their life and I hope to help you too. Even if you just have a few rough nights, there is no need to be frightened. I always find it more comforting to know what is going on with my body, and then I am not frightened. I want to empower you.

*I am starting to go through the changes of menopause and my friends say that I will never sleep again?*

**Yes, you will sleep again**, with these Vital Tools:

Read the following statements every day and try to replace your current thoughts and beliefs about your sleep with these statements below.

Even if you do not believe all this right now----consider the following…. Is what you are doing and believing working for you? If not, give yourself 8 WEEKS, follow these directions as best you can, suspend your beliefs and pretend to believe what I am telling you to believe below----read this list out loud to yourself every day!

## Sleeping Well!

1.     The most important behavioral change that I can make is to get up at the same time everyday regardless of how much I have slept the night before. This will help keep my circadian clock on track. I will set my alarm and **turn my clock around**.

2.     I will use my bed only for sleeping and sex. I will not read, eat, watch TV, or do any other distracting things in my bed.

3.     If I have a bad night when I can't sleep and I have been awake long enough to be bothered by it, I'll just get out of bed and go in another room and do something relaxing (like watching TV or listening to music) until I feel sleepy again. I will not turn on any bright lights. Use a night light or small flashlight. Then when I feel sleepy again, I will go back to my bed and fall asleep.

4.     Early each evening, I will make a "To Do List" for the next day and even sit down and journal any things that are bothering me. I will not worry or plan when I lay down to go to bed at night.

5.     Napping is fine for people when they do not have any problems sleeping at night. However, napping, particularly in the afternoon or evening will interfere with my nighttime sleep so I do not want to do that now.

6.     **I will go to bed only when I am sleepy**, but in order to consolidate my sleep I am not going to go to bed earlier than the time suggested by my **"sleep consolidator"**.

7.     I will get out in **bright light in the morning** and avoid bright light at night. That means shutting off my computer at least 2 hours before my bedtime!

## Major helpful hints:

1.     Make your bedroom quiet, dark, and cool. **60-67 degrees** is suggested by the National Sleep Foundation.

2.     Consider using a floor or window fan to both drowned out intermittent noises that may arouse you through the night as well as be a modality for cooling. Put your feet in the breeze of a fan if you awaken and are warm or have a hot flash.

3.     Limit caffeine---none after 12 noon.

4.     No alcohol after ~7 PM. Even though alcohol can make you sleepy, once it is metabolized (~ 3 hours) it will wake you and contribute to disrupted sleep.

5.     Avoid the steady use of sleeping pills.

6.     **Exercise regularly** but not within 3 hours of going to bed. Exercise raises your core body temperature and that makes it hard to fall asleep and stay asleep. Remember, we fall asleep as our body temperature drops, and we stay asleep as

long as our temperature stays cool. We wake when it rises.

7.    Schedule some quiet time before bed to wind down. Get away from the computer and the smartphone and avoid bright light at night.

8.    Some people benefit from a light snack such as milk,  a bite of peanut butter, or a piece of cheese so as not to wake from hunger in the night. But make sure it is a light snack. Eating more will aggravate acid reflux and cause weight gain.

Now the minimum time in bed for sleep is 5 ½ hours in bed. Most people are actually sleeping more than they think and **within 2 weeks should be able to expand their time in bed to a more reasonable 6-7 hours**. It may come as a surprise to some, but the odds of becoming excessively sleepy following sleep restriction or consolidation treatment was not different from that of being nonsleepy. (22)

The second most common trap that women fall into is Sleep State Misperception. We now understand we will wake at this time of our lives due to rising temperature. When we wake, the common behavior is to look at the clock. Remember that we have amnesia for about 5 minutes before we fall asleep. Well, this is how we misinterpret waking from sleeping. If we wake at 2 AM and look at the clock and make note of the time and then we fall back asleep but just into light sleep (normal sleep is comprised of 60% light sleep). Then wake again and look at the clock and make note of the time and it is 2:30 AM, we do not realize we slept, and we get angry and frustrated, which is not helping the situation. We may be up longer but drift off and then wake again at 3 AM and look at the clock and when this repeats over and over, we will not feel that we have slept at all, but we have slept. I created this in my own sleep, and I have always been a particularly good sleeper. I was amazed at how easy this distortion can occur.

Remember, it is normal to take up to 30 minutes to fall asleep. But the more we get upset about this, raising our alertness, the less we are able to appreciate any intervening sleep. It feels as though we have not slept but we may have slept and just not known it because we have amnesia for the time around falling asleep. Unless we had a dream (which implies deeper sleep) we will not know that we slept. I am not saying that everyone who feels they are not sleeping has this, but this is a common pitfall. This is the reason that I emphasize having you set your alarm and turn your clock around, so that you will not watch the clock. This is also the reason why it is suggested to get out of bed when you are not sleeping and go into another room. You want to differentiate sleep from wake and associate your bed only with sleeping.

Have you ever been lying there in bed frustrated, thinking, "I haven't slept" and then remembered or realized a ridiculous or weird dream? Only then do you question yourself to think, "*I must have fallen asleep*". Has anyone ever said to you, you were sleeping or snoring when you thought you were awake all night? This is an example of Sleep State Misperception. You are not telling a lie; it is a misperception. You feel awake and not rested. That, however, does not mean you did not sleep.

So again, I want to optimize your chances of a good sleep. To do this we have already reviewed that your body sleeps best when trying to sleep on its natural circadian rhythm. But most of us must conform to a certain schedule for work and for our family's schedule. If that is not the same schedule as our circadian rhythm, then what do we do? Well, I want you to know that you can change your internal rhythm just like people do with jetlag and travelling over different time zones. The key to remember here is that your rhythm is set by the time you get up every day and by light!

So, by getting up every day at the same time, no matter if you slept or not and getting bright light at that time for approximately 30 minutes you can change your rhythm! It takes about 2 weeks to get your new rhythm trained and working. However, if you sleep in even just one morning, your body will revert to its natural (old) rhythm and you must start all over again.

Now if your desired wake up time is less than 3 hours away from your current and natural (days off) wake up time---go ahead and set this. Set your alarm and turn your clock around! No peeking at your smartphone either! Back out your average hours of sleep (not what you want, but what you counted on your sleep logs) and add 30 minutes. This is your **_sleep consolidator_**. Now if this gives you less than 5½ hours, I want you to use 5 ½ hours as your time in bed. So if you want to set your sleep rhythm to get up at 7 AM, and you do not think that you have been sleeping even 5 ½ hours each night, you would set your bedtime to 1:30 AM. Continue your sleep logs while you are on this schedule and you will start to see how your sleep starts to consolidate. Now it is normal to wake through the night and take up to 30 minutes to fall back asleep. Most good sleepers do not remember waking because they do not focus on it. Remember, you have amnesia for the time you fall asleep and approximately 5 minutes beforehand. So, if you wake, turn over, arrange your pillow and fall back asleep you probably will not remember it --- unless you became angry and frustrated with waking or taking more than 5 minutes to fall back asleep. This can easily happen with hot flashes because it is hard to cool off that fast. Remember your "thermal inertia" may take 25-100 minutes for your core body temperature to drop. But just realizing that it is the hot flash or your body temperature that is waking you, *knowing* that you can do some things to facilitate cooling your body like putting your feet in the cool breeze of the fan, a cold compress on your forehead, and kicking off the covers,...*can empower you* with *both the knowledge of what is going on and some techniques* to combat these sleep disruptions. You can remedy what is happening to your body. And ...*it is not that anything is wrong with your brain*...

So, what if you are on an odd schedule? How do you shift your circadian rhythm? Remember I said there was one caveat to this simple method of changing your circadian rhythm---if your new wake up time is more than 3 hours earlier than your natural rhythm: you must move your wake-up time back 1 hour per week for a few weeks to reach your desired wake up time. This is due to a special physiology that occurs 3 hours before your natural wake up time. So, moving your wake-up time back 3 hours or more all at once will paradoxically give you the opposite result.

Do the same technique but just move the wake-up time back one hour each week----Set your alarm and turn your clock around! No peeking at your smartphone. Back out your average hours of sleep (not what you want, but what you counted on your sleep logs) and add 30 minutes. This is your "*sleep consolidator*". Again, if this gives you less than 5 ½ hours, it is important to use the minimum of 5 ½ hours as your time in bed.

Continue your sleep logs while you are on this schedule and you will start to see how your sleep starts to consolidate. Now it is normal to wake through the night and take up to 30 minutes to fall back asleep. Remember your "thermal inertia" may take 25-100 minutes for your core body temperature to drop.

Now, you may ask, how do I fill out my sleep logs if I cannot see the clock? Good question. I want you to fill out the log in the morning based on what you remember about your sleep the night before, and the fuzzier it is, the better. Our aim is to decrease your alertness during the night, not increase it. You know what time you went to bed and what time you got out of bed in the morning. That is sufficient. The rest can be estimated.

Key points to remember; *the <u>same wake-up time every day</u>* and *<u>keep cool!</u>* Add exercise and you have my mantra- the *3T's to get your Z's*....<u>Timing</u>, <u>Temperature</u> and the <u>Track</u>!

It was demonstrated in a simple randomized controlled trial that even light-intensity walking improved how fast the older women with mild sleep impairment fall asleep and improved their sleep efficiency (23).

Lastly, after all that I have said above if your hot flashes are too severe do not be afraid to ask your gynecologist for help with short term medication. Also, if you are working hard to consolidate your sleep and you have had more than 4 really tough nights; it is ok to take an over the counter sleep aid or prescription sleep aid once per week for *a short time* to catch up if you don't have a medical contraindication to this; but this should be done on only *one or two scheduled nights* and I typically suggest this for Sunday night to help you start your week.

Once you are sleeping 90% of the time that you are in bed, which may only be 5 hours if you are in bed 5 ½ hours, then you can add 15-30 minutes to your allotted time in bed, usually by going to bed 15-30 minutes earlier, because you want to keep your wake-up time steady. This same step can be repeated over and over until you have expanded your sleep with your time in bed to meet your sleep needs, as long as you are sleeping most of the time you are in bed.

I want you to sleep as much as your body needs as long as it is fairly consolidated. There is no "one size fits all" and your sleep may vary slightly with the seasons. It is naturally light earlier in the morning, and daylight lasts later into the evening in the summer. This light difference may affect how much sleep you need or get. Also, exercise and medications may change the amount of sleep you get naturally.

Importantly, *if you have not slept well and are sleepy, do not drive! Driving sleepy is the same as driving drunk*. Carpool or ask for a ride. You would do the same for a friend.

Remember the three T's to get your Z's....*Timing, Temperature and the Track!*

# SLEEP AFTER MENOPAUSE

So now you have the tools to understand what is happening to your sleep during this change in your life. This is not a permanent blow to your ability to sleep unless you "learn" how to perpetuate bad sleep. You can refuse to "learn" bad sleep and keep reminding yourself how your body sleeps best and enhance that in every way possible. Try to keep a sense of humor: this will not last forever. Please get help if or when you need it. Keep your body cool! Use a fan, a cool cloth on your forehead, a refrigerated gel pack for your forehead, neck, or whatever works for you. And this sleep disruption caused by fluctuating hormones will improve, as your hormones level out. So, do not "learn" another sleep problem to turn into chronic insomnia while you are dealing with a *temporary* situation with your hormone changes. The hormone change is permanent, but the *SLOPE of the change* is what is causing you the major disruption and that ***dramatic change is temporary***.

Do not be discouraged if you are doing well and then all the sudden things get disrupted. Go through the things that you know to do, and it will reset again. Remember, this is like a staircase, if you are lucky, there will be step-downs with symptoms and then plateaus. Keep these tools and pull them out whenever you need them. There are additional AASM sleep diaries/logs and an extra copy of the **"Sleeping Well!" and "Major helpful hints"** included at the end of this book for your easy reference any time you need them. Remember to keep your wake-up time steady, at least within a one-hour timeframe between workdays and days off, keep cool, even cooler than you would normally choose. Many women, like myself, have been cold most of their life and their habit has been to dress warm and cozy to relax in the evening. It feels odd to change the sleeping environment to be so cold. But I now set my furnace to drop to 60 degrees F at 11 PM in the winter. I am a fan of all cotton sheets and sleeping with minimal or no clothing to help keep cool and to keep from getting tangled up when shifting positions. I suggest layering your covers with a light cotton sheet, then a light blanket and finally a comforter, so that you can start out with the covers needed and throw them off or pull them up as you cycle through different temperatures. I suggest a dimmer on your light switches or a three level light bulb in your bedside lamp so that you can turn down the covers and dim the lights when you are getting ready for bed and avoid having to turn on any bright lights. Turning on the fan can even be a sonic cue for sleep. You can do this even well before you are ready to go to bed so that the room is ready when you decide to go to bed. Get regular exercise but not close to bedtime, remember not within 3 hours of bedtime because it heats up your core body temperature. And do not go to bed until you are sleepy. When you are sleeping well, sleep as much as your body needs to feel good. ***Be kind to yourself in this process. Remember it is a process!*** Get help from a sleep specialist if you try these methods but do not get good results or if you have concerns about some of the sleep disorders that I reviewed and their symptoms as these are common problems that can be treated effectively.

Please feel free to share comments with me on how I might improve this learning process. Tell me what helped you most and what you did not find helpful. You can send your comments to me at my website; www.agoodnightssleep.net. I wish you best of health and happiness.

Remember my mantra—
# The 3T's to get your Z's...
## *Timing, Temperature, and the Track!*

And now, for the bonus chapter, the treat that you have all been waiting for... I'd like to introduce the "only other activity that is important besides sleep in the bedroom---"sex" by my friend and colleague...

# SEX AFTER MENOPAUSE
by Marcia Klein-Patel, M.D., PhD

Why does a book about sleep have a chapter about sex? Besides the fact that sex is the only other activity recommended for the bedroom other than sleep... It is because in our clinical practice, we commonly have patients present with concerns about sleep and sex. In some ways they are interdependent.

As Dr. Sunseri has stressed before, all healthy living can be reduced to eating well, exercising, having good relationships, and sleeping well. However, have you ever noticed how hard it is to have the first three if you do not have the last? It is impossibly hard to have headspace to think about intimacy, let alone maintain a satisfying relationship, if you are fatigued, stressed about sleep and the worried about the next day.

When I begin to evaluate a patient for sexual concerns, I think about it in three parts:
1) sexual function 2) changes in the vulva and vagina and 3) health and lifestyle factors. How we can address these issues will be discussed at the end of the chapter.

What is normal sexual function?
**Normal sexual function is defined by you**! There is no set frequency, duration, or type of intimacy that defines normal. If you are comfortable with your level of sexual desire, response, and function then that is normal. In general, experts would say that normal sexual function includes some degree of desire and an ability to enjoy sex. Additionally, *if you are not bothered then there is no problem*. And while many couples report satisfying intimacy their entire relationships, about 33-50% of peri- and postmenopausal women will describe some level of bother.

There are **three Phases of Sexual Response.** Sexual response in women has been extensively written about and can be thought of in 3 major components: **Desire, arousal,** and **response and pleasure.** Desire is the biologic component that manifests itself as sexual thoughts and fantasies. It can be affected by one's personal attitudes toward sex and can wax and wane throughout the lifespan and relationship. *Motivation for intimacy* is a complex and important part of desire as well. If someone reports *distress secondary to decreased desire*, then it *becomes a concern.* Hypoactive sexual desire disorder includes by definition the lack of fantasies or thoughts and lack of desire for sexual activity, *and this causes the person personal distress.*

**One in three women report decreased desire.** Causes of decreased desire in women are *multifactorial.* As noted above, **conflicts with the partner, medical problems, or culture beliefs** will impact desire. Studies note that women tend to be more bothered if they are in a relationship, are between 35-64 years of age, or are depressed. Happiness in one's relationship has a positive impact on desire!

*Arousal* encompasses the physical signs of sexual readiness. These include increased blood flow to the vulva, vagina, and clitoris as well as increased lubrication. ***Changes in hormone levels and vaginal changes can affect arousal.*** This is more common in women in midlife (approximately 7.5%) and may be exacerbated in women who have had early surgical menopause.

Last, but not least, ***response and pleasure*** are the culmination of fulfilling the desire and arousal stages. However, some women report that the changes in blood flow and decreased sensitivity of the clitoris can affect orgasm. They may report it is less intense, may take longer to achieve, or they may lose the ability to consistently achieve orgasm.

Changes in the vulva and vagina are the most common, but not the only physical change women bring to their gynecologists' attention. Genital syndrome of menopause, previously called vulvovaginal atrophy, is a result of decreased estrogen, which causes the vagina to become thinner, drier, and less flexible. The rugae (or folds) of the vagina flatten out, making distensibility more difficult. This is the most common cause of painful sex for women over the age of 50. Between 17 and 45% of postmenopausal women report that sex is painful for them. Fortunately, regular intercourse can preserve thickness and moisture of tissues, and help maintain vaginal caliber. Unfortunately, infrequent use can result in the vagina becoming shorter and narrower and can result in anxiety regarding future intimacy, arousal, and involuntary tightening of the vaginal muscles.

I also always ensure to evaluate other causes of vulvar and vaginal pain. We frequently see vulvar dermatosis as the cause of painful intercourse. Causes include contact dermatitis (as can be seen in chronic pad use for urinary leakage), yeast infections secondary to medications or diabetes, autoimmune changes to the vulva which leave it fragile and less commonly vulvar cancer. If you or your partner notice changes of the vulvar skin, it is important to have those followed up by your gynecologist.

Lastly, the muscles of the pelvic floor can spasm also leading to painful intercourse. These can be seen after birth trauma, with orthopedic injuries, or bowel disturbances. It is crowded in the pelvis! If one tissue is out of balance, it can set the whole pelvic area out of balance. Sometimes, positioning can make the difference and the pain only occurs with some types of activity. It is always useful to be honest with your gynecologist and bring these issues to the attention of your provider to help solve any underlying issues.

**What else can affect sex after menopause?** Well, we are complex human beings. There are a lot of factors that affect how we function. Our overall health and our lifestyle have a lot to do with how we function.

First, if you or your partner are having significant health concerns, these concerns will supersede the desire to have intimacy. In many cases, this is rightly so. This includes things such as cancer, diabetes, hypertension, and mood changes in you or your partner. Inattention to these matters may worsen sexual function in the future (as well as your sleep). They may also affect your self-image which may further impact sexual function. It is important to work with a provider you trust to reach your best health.

Think about your day. Are you exercising? Are you working every moment of the day, either in or out of the home? Are you caring for grown children? Aging parents? Is the last thing that you think about as you go to your room the work that still needs to be done? Or are you thinking about the refreshing sleep you are about to have, either before or after you have sex? Do you and your partner have the same sleep/wake cycles? So many couples work opposite hours from each other, hardly ever seeing each other. It is important to make sex an equal priority to the other things on our "to do" list.

Lastly, evaluate the communication in your relationship. Is it a safe place where you each feel supported? You cannot have intimacy if you do not like your partner. (Well, unless you get a new partner).

**Effective treatments for sexual concerns are available!**
First and foremost, talk with your provider.

Some sexual problems may signal underlying medical problems. Effective treatments often combine multiple modalities and there is no need for you and your partner to suffer in silence. If you are having difficulty finding a provider in your area you can check with the provider listings at the North American Menopause Society. Their website is https://www.menopause.org. The International Society for the Study of Women's Sexual Health is another good source. Their website is https://www.isswsh.org.

The *importance of lifestyle* cannot be overstated. Again, exercising regularly (not too close to bedtime), maintaining a healthy weight, eating right, smoking cessation, moderation in alcohol use, adequate regular sleep and regular stimulation all improve sexual function. There are no shortcuts.

Some couples may find that in order to restore health sexual relations, they may need to resolve broader issues. *Both relationship and sex therapy may be helpful* in these instances. Sex therapists are mental health providers who use a targeted approach to talk about sexual feelings openly. They may involve strategies to improve intimacy such as sensate focused exercises.

For women with vulvar vaginal discomfort, it is useful to start with topical treatments. Our first choice is always lubricants. For some couples this may be new to them, but in our office, we say, "*lube for life*!" Lubricants should be used with every sexual act. In general, for people who have not yet tried lubricants, we recommend **water-based first**, you can find them everywhere (grocery store, pharmacy, and internet). Sometimes, you may need to try several until you find one that you like. Adult stores and internet specialty shops will often sell trial packs. Some women have more success with silicone-based lubricants as they can be silkier and last a little longer. Often your local retailer may sell one or two, but they can be readily found on the internet. In general, we tend to avoid oil-based lubricants as they can break down condoms and about 30% of postmenopausal women will find them irritating. If you are using one and it works for you – that is great!

**Moisturizers** are also useful in the treatment of

the genital syndrome of menopause. They act *just as moisturizers do on other body parts*, by holding in water. These are not used at the time of intercourse but a couple of times a week. Just as you might apply a special moisturizing facial cream before bed, think about applying a special moisturizer for your vagina!

So, it is prudent to consider using both a lubricant and a moisturizer. Lastly, for women without contraindications, there are *prescription topical estrogen-based products* that can be helpful. These all are worth a discussion with your health care provider and are generally very safe and well tolerated. The mode of delivery can vary. This may come as a cream with an applicator to insert it in your vagina. Systemic hormones, that is those taken by mouth, and other prescriptions used for libido should be carefully reviewed with your health care provider to weigh their risks verses their benefits.

*Examples of commonly used lubricants, moisturizers, and vaginal estrogen products* are listed in the table on the next page and there is an extra copy in the back of the book for you to tear out and keep in your purse to have with you when you go to the pharmacy or to discuss with your doctor.

## Examples of commonly used lubricants, moisturizers, and vaginal estrogen products

| | |
|---|---|
| **Lubricants** | *Water-based:* Good Clean Love, Astroglide, FemGlide, Just Like Me, K-Y Jelly, Pre-Seed, Slippery Stuff, Summer's Eve, others <br> *Silicone-based:* Uber lube, ID Millennium, Pink, Pjur, Pure Pleasure, others <br> *Oil-based (avoid with condoms):* Coconut oil, Olive oil, Mineral oil, Elegance Woman's Lubricant, others |
| **Vaginal moisturizers** | Fresh Start, K-Y Silk-E, Moist Again, Replens, K-Y Liquibeads, Good Clean Love, others |
| **Vaginal estrogen products** | Vagifem (vaginal tablet), Estrace (cream), Neo-Estrone (cream), Premarin (cream), Estring (low-dose vaginal ring), Osphena (ospemifene, pill) |

Other adjuncts to pelvic health can include **pelvic yoga** which can improve self-image, relaxation and pelvic floor strengthening. **Kegel exercises** can improve urinary incontinence, increase muscle awareness, and reduce pain with sex. In patients with poor muscular control or hyperactive muscles we will often recommend pelvic floor physical therapy with biofeedback either with a therapist or with a biofeedback device.

Additionally, our behaviors will affect our frequency and enjoyment of intercourse. Activities like **reading "sexy" books**, scheduling **date nights**, and experimenting with different positions, toys or other play can all improve desire. There are many good resources online and your neighborhood adult shop can also be helpful. **Vibrators and positioning pillows can be a useful tool** to a healthy sex life. Other devices such as **clitoral stimulation devices** (FDA approved devices like Eros and Fiera) may also be recommended by your provider.

Even though sexual issues are common in women and sexual function in women can be complex, effective treatments and therapies exist. It is important to find a provider with whom you are comfortable discussing these issues. Do not ignore the impact of the mind, body, and spirit. Through addressing any concerns you have, understanding that you are a complex and beautiful human being, I hope you can find validation that although complex, you have options and treatments and you can find the right approach that works for you.

## TWO WEEK SLEEP DIARY

INSTRUCTIONS:
1. Write the date, day of the week, and type of day: Work, School, Day Off, or Vacation.
2. Put the letter "C" in the box when you have coffee, cola or tea. Put "M" when you take any medicine. Put "A" when you drink alcohol. Put "E" when you exercise.
3. Put a line (I) to show when you go to bed. Shade in the box that shows when you think you fell asleep.
4. Shade in all the boxes that show when you are asleep at night or when you take a nap during the day.
5. Leave boxes unshaded to show when you wake up at night and when you are awake during the day.

SAMPLE ENTRY BELOW: On a Monday when I worked, I jogged on my lunch break at 1 PM, had a glass of wine with dinner at 6 PM, fell asleep watching TV from 7 to 8 PM, went to bed at 10:30 PM, fell asleep around Midnight, woke up and couldn't got back to sleep at about 4 AM, went back to sleep from 5 to 7 AM, and had coffee and medicine at 7:00 in the morning.

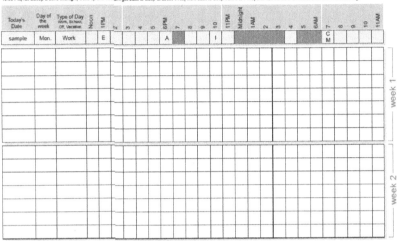

## TWO WEEK SLEEP DIARY

INSTRUCTIONS:
1. Write the date, day of the week, and type of day: Work, School, Day Off, or Vacation.
2. Put the letter "C" in the box when you have coffee, cola or tea. Put "M" when you take any medicine. Put "A" when you drink alcohol. Put "E" when you exercise.
3. Put a line (I) to show when you go to bed. Shade in the box that shows when you think you fell asleep.
4. Shade in all the boxes that show when you are asleep at night or when you take a nap during the day.
5. Leave boxes unshaded to show when you wake up at night and when you are awake during the day.

SAMPLE ENTRY BELOW: On a Monday when I worked, I jogged on my lunch break at 1 PM, had a glass of wine with dinner at 6 PM, fell asleep watching TV from 7 to 8 PM, went to bed at 10:30 PM, fell asleep around Midnight, woke up and couldn't got back to sleep at about 4 AM, went back to sleep from 5 to 7 AM, and had coffee and medicine at 7:00 in the morning.

# M. J. Sunseri, M.D.

## TWO WEEK SLEEP DIARY

INSTRUCTIONS:
1. Write the date, day of the week, and type of day: Work, School, Day Off, or Vacation.
2. Put the letter "C" in the box when you have coffee, cola or tea. Put "M" when you take any medicine. Put "A" when you drink alcohol. Put "E" when you exercise.
3. Put a line (I) to show when you go to bed. Shade in the box that shows when you think you fell asleep.
4. Shade in all the boxes that show when you are asleep at night or when you take a nap during the day.
5. Leave boxes unshaded to show when you wake up at night and when you are awake during the day.

SAMPLE ENTRY BELOW: On a Monday when I worked, I jogged on my lunch break at 1 PM, had a glass of wine with dinner at 6 PM, fell asleep watching TV from 7 to 8 PM, went to bed at 10:30 PM, fell asleep around Midnight, woke up and couldn't get back to sleep at about 4 AM, went back to sleep from 5 to 7 AM, and had coffee and medicine at 7:00 in the morning.

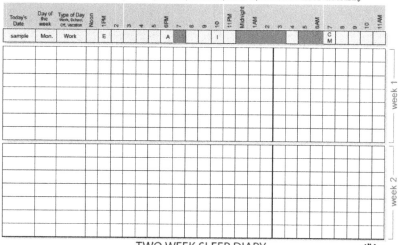

## TWO WEEK SLEEP DIARY

INSTRUCTIONS:
1. Write the date, day of the week, and type of day: Work, School, Day Off, or Vacation.
2. Put the letter "C" in the box when you have coffee, cola or tea. Put "M" when you take any medicine. Put "A" when you drink alcohol. Put "E" when you exercise.
3. Put a line (I) to show when you go to bed. Shade in the box that shows when you think you fell asleep.
4. Shade in all the boxes that show when you are asleep at night or when you take a nap during the day.
5. Leave boxes unshaded to show when you wake up at night and when you are awake during the day.

SAMPLE ENTRY BELOW: On a Monday when I worked, I jogged on my lunch break at 1 PM, had a glass of wine with dinner at 6 PM, fell asleep watching TV from 7 to 8 PM, went to bed at 10:30 PM, fell asleep around Midnight, woke up and couldn't get back to sleep at about 4 AM, went back to sleep from 5 to 7 AM, and had coffee and medicine at 7:00 in the morning.

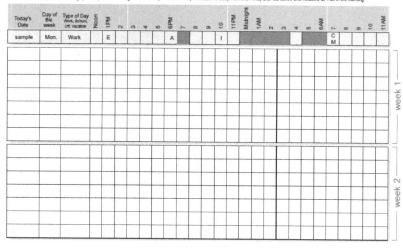

## TWO WEEK SLEEP DIARY

INSTRUCTIONS:
1. Write the date, day of the week, and type of day: Work, School, Day Off, or Vacation.
2. Put the letter "C" in the box when you have coffee, cola or tea. Put "M" when you take any medicine. Put "A" when you drink alcohol. Put "E" when you exercise.
3. Put a line (I) to show when you go to bed. Shade in the box that shows when you think you fell asleep.
4. Shade in all the boxes that show when you are asleep at night or when you take a nap during the day.
5. Leave boxes unshaded to show when you wake up at night and when you are awake during the day.

SAMPLE ENTRY BELOW: On a Monday when I worked, I jogged on my lunch break at 1 PM, had a glass of wine with dinner at 6 PM, fell asleep watching TV from 7 to 8 PM, went to bed at 10:30 PM, fell asleep around Midnight, woke up and couldn't got back to sleep at about 4 AM, went back to sleep from 5 to 7 AM, and had coffee and medicine at 7:00 in the morning.

| Today's Date | Day of the week | Type of Day Work, School, Off, Vacation | Noon | 1PM | 2 | 3 | 4 | 5 | 6PM | 7 | 8 | 9 | 10 | 11PM | Midnight | 1AM | 2 | 3 | 4 | 5 | 6AM | 7 | 8 | 9 | 10 | 11AM |
|---|---|---|---|---|---|---|---|---|---|---|---|---|---|---|---|---|---|---|---|---|---|---|---|---|---|---|
| sample | Mon. | Work | E | | | | | | A | | | | | | I | | | | | | | C M | | | | |

week 1

week 2

## TWO WEEK SLEEP DIARY

INSTRUCTIONS:
1. Write the date, day of the week, and type of day: Work, School, Day Off, or Vacation.
2. Put the letter "C" in the box when you have coffee, cola or tea. Put "M" when you take any medicine. Put "A" when you drink alcohol. Put "E" when you exercise.
3. Put a line (I) to show when you go to bed. Shade in the box that shows when you think you fell asleep.
4. Shade in all the boxes that show when you are asleep at night or when you take a nap during the day.
5. Leave boxes unshaded to show when you wake up at night and when you are awake during the day.

SAMPLE ENTRY BELOW: On a Monday when I worked, I jogged on my lunch break at 1 PM, had a glass of wine with dinner at 6 PM, fell asleep watching TV from 7 to 8 PM, went to bed at 10:30 PM, fell asleep around Midnight, woke up and couldn't got back to sleep at about 4 AM, went back to sleep from 5 to 7 AM, and had coffee and medicine at 7:00 in the morning.

| Today's Date | Day of the week | Type of Day Work, School, Off, Vacation | Noon | 1PM | 2 | 3 | 4 | 5 | 6PM | 7 | 8 | 9 | 10 | 11PM | Midnight | 1AM | 2 | 3 | 4 | 5 | 6AM | 7 | 8 | 9 | 10 | 11AM |
|---|---|---|---|---|---|---|---|---|---|---|---|---|---|---|---|---|---|---|---|---|---|---|---|---|---|---|
| sample | Mon. | Work | E | | | | | | A | | | | | | I | | | | | | | C M | | | | |

week 1

week 2

# M. J. Sunseri, M.D.

## TWO WEEK SLEEP DIARY

**INSTRUCTIONS:**
1. Write the date, day of the week, and type of day: Work, School, Day Off, or Vacation.
2. Put the letter "C" in the box when you have coffee, cola or tea. Put "M" when you take any medicine. Put "A" when you drink alcohol. Put "E" when you exercise.
3. Put a line (l) to show when you go to bed. Shade in the box that shows when you think you fell asleep.
4. Shade in all the boxes that show when you are asleep at night or when you take a nap during the day.
5. Leave boxes unshaded to show when you wake up at night and when you are awake during the day.

*SAMPLE ENTRY BELOW:* On a Monday when I worked, I jogged on my lunch break at 1 PM, had a glass of wine with dinner at 6 PM, fell asleep watching TV from 7 to 8 PM, went to bed at 10:30 PM, fell asleep around Midnight, woke up and couldn't get back to sleep at about 4 AM, went back to sleep from 5 to 7 AM, and had coffee and medicine at 7:00 in the morning.

| Today's Date | Day of the week | Type of Day Work, School, Off, Vacation | Noon | 1 PM | 2 | 3 | 4 | 5 | 6PM | 7 | 8 | 9 | 10 | 11PM | Midnight | 1 AM | 2 | 3 | 4 | 5 | 6AM | 7 | 8 | 9 | 10 | 11 PM | |
|---|---|---|---|---|---|---|---|---|---|---|---|---|---|---|---|---|---|---|---|---|---|---|---|---|---|---|---|
| sample | Mon. | Work | | E | | | | | A | | | | | | I | | | | | | C M | | | | | | |
| | | | | | | | | | | | | | | | | | | | | | | | | | | | | week 1 |
| | | | | | | | | | | | | | | | | | | | | | | | | | | | | week 2 |

## TWO WEEK SLEEP DIARY

**INSTRUCTIONS:**
1. Write the date, day of the week, and type of day: Work, School, Day Off, or Vacation.
2. Put the letter "C" in the box when you have coffee, cola or tea. Put "M" when you take any medicine. Put "A" when you drink alcohol. Put "E" when you exercise.
3. Put a line (l) to show when you go to bed. Shade in the box that shows when you think you fell asleep.
4. Shade in all the boxes that show when you are asleep at night or when you take a nap during the day.
5. Leave boxes unshaded to show when you wake up at night and when you are awake during the day.

*SAMPLE ENTRY BELOW:* On a Monday when I worked, I jogged on my lunch break at 1 PM, had a glass of wine with dinner at 6 PM, fell asleep watching TV from 7 to 8 PM, went to bed at 10:30 PM, fell asleep around Midnight, woke up and couldn't get back to sleep at about 4 AM, went back to sleep from 5 to 7 AM, and had coffee and medicine at 7:00 in the morning.

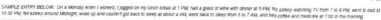

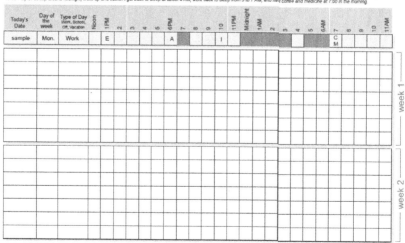

| Today's Date | Day of the week | Type of Day Work, School, Off, Vacation | Noon | 1PM | 2 | 3 | 4 | 5 | 6PM | 7 | 8 | 9 | 10 | 11PM | Midnight | 1AM | 2 | 3 | 4 | 5 | 6AM | 7 | 8 | 9 | 10 | 11AM | |
|---|---|---|---|---|---|---|---|---|---|---|---|---|---|---|---|---|---|---|---|---|---|---|---|---|---|---|---|
| sample | Mon. | Work | | E | | | | | A | | | | | | I | | | | | | C M | | | | | | |
| | | | | | | | | | | | | | | | | | | | | | | | | | | | | week 1 |
| | | | | | | | | | | | | | | | | | | | | | | | | | | | | week 2 |

## <u>Sleeping Well!</u>

1.      The most important behavioral change that I can make is to get up at the same time everyday regardless of how much I have slept the night before. This will help keep my circadian clock on track. I will set my alarm and **turn my clock around**.

2.      I will use my bed only for sleeping and sex. I will not read, eat, watch TV or do any other distracting things in my bed.

3.      If I have a bad night when I can't sleep and I have been awake long enough to be bothered by it, I'll just get out of bed and go in another room and do something relaxing (like listening to music) until I feel sleepy again. **I will not turn on any bright lights.** Use a night light or small flashlight. Then when I feel sleepy again, I'll go back to my bed and fall asleep.

4.      Early each evening I will make a **"To Do List"** for the next day and even sit down and journal any things that are bothering me. I will not worry or plan when I lay down to go to bed at night.

5.      Napping is fine for people when they do not have any problems sleeping at night. However, napping, particularly in the afternoon or evening will interfere with my nighttime sleep so I do not want to do that now.

6.      I will go to bed only when I am sleepy, but in order to consolidate my sleep I am not going to go to bed earlier than the time suggested by my sleep consolidator.

7.      I will get out in **bright light in the morning** and avoid bright light at night. That means shutting off my computer at least 2 hours before my bedtime!

## <u>Major helpful hints:</u>

1)      Make your bedroom quiet, dark and cool. **60-67degrees** is suggested by the National Sleep Foundation.

2)      Consider using a floor or window fan to both drowned out intermittent noises that may arouse you through the night as well as be a modality for cooling your feet if you awaken and are warm or have a hot flash.

3)      Limit caffeine---none after 12 noon.

4)      No alcohol after ~7 PM. Even though alcohol can make you sleepy, once it is metabolized (~ 3 hours) it will wake you and contribute to disrupted sleep.

5)      Avoid the steady use of sleeping pills.

6)      Exercise regularly but not within 3 hours of going to bed.  Exercise raises your core body temperature and that makes it hard to fall asleep and stay asleep.

7)      Schedule some quiet time before bed to wind down. Get away from the computer and the smart phone and **avoid bright light**.

8)      Some people benefit from a light snack such as milk, peanut butter or a piece of cheese so as not to wake from hunger in the night. But make sure it is a **light** snack. Eating more will aggravate acid reflux and cause weight gain.

| Examples of commonly used lubricants, moisturizers, and vaginal estrogen products | |
| --- | --- |
| **Lubricants** | *Water-based:* Good Clean Love, Astroglide, FemGlide, Just Like Me, K-Y Jelly, Pre-Seed, Slippery Stuff, Summer's Eve, others<br>*Silicone-based:* Uber lube, ID Millennium, Pink, Pjur, Pure Pleasure, others<br>*Oil-based (avoid with condoms):* Coconut oil, Olive oil, Mineral oil, Elegance Woman's Lubricant, others |
| **Vaginal moisturizers** | Fresh Start, K-Y Silk-E, Moist Again, Replens, K-Y Liquibeads, Good Clean Love, others |
| **Vaginal estrogen products** | Vagifem (vaginal tablet), Estrace (cream), Neo-Estrone (cream), Premarin (cream), Estring (low-dose vaginal ring), Osphena (ospemifene, pill) |

# ABOUT THE AUTHOR

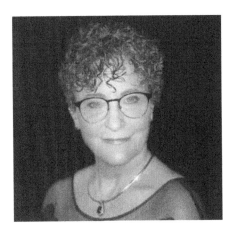

Dr. Sunseri is a board-certified neurologist specializing in sleep disorders, including women's sleep disorders, and their connection to other conditions and illnesses.

She completed her undergraduate studies in biochemistry/biophysics at the University of Pittsburgh and earned her medical degree from the University of Pittsburgh, School of Medicine. She completed a general medical internship at Riverside Methodist Hospital in Columbus, Ohio, and completed her residency in neurology at Georgetown University Hospital, Washington, D.C.

Dr. Sunseri completed a sleep medicine research fellowship at Cliniques Saint-Luc, University of Louvain, Brussels, Belgium.

Dr. Sunseri is certified by the American Board of Psychiatry and Neurology with an additional subspecialty certification in Clinical Neurophysiology. She also is certified by the American Board of Medical Specialties subspecializing in Sleep Medicine. Other certifications include the American Board of Sleep Medicine and the American Board of Clinical Neurophysiology.

Her professional affiliations include the American Academy of Neurology, Pennsylvania Medical Society, Allegheny County Medical Society, and she is a Fellow with the American Academy of Sleep Medicine.

Dr. Sunseri has participated in medical research and clinical trials, has given countless presentations and lectures. She has published book chapters and scientific articles but has been most excited to publish this book for women of all backgrounds to guide them at this important juncture in their lives.

# REFERENCES:

1    Dimitrov, S. et al. Sleep associated regulation of T helper 1/T helper 2 cytokine balance in humans. Brain, Behavior and Immunity 18 (2004) 341-348.

2    Besedovsky, L. et al. Sleep and immune function. Invited Review. Pflugers Arch-Eur J Physiol (2012) 463:121-137.

3    Lulu Xie, Hongyi Kang, Qiwu Xu, Michael J.Chen, Yonghong Liao, Meenakshisundaram Thiyagarajan, John O'Donnell, Daniel J. Christensen, Charles Nicholson, Jeffrey J. Iliff, Takahiro Takano, Rashid Deane, and Maiken Nedergaard. Sleep Drives Metabolite Clearance from the Adult Brain. Science 2013 October 18; 342 (6156)

4    Nathaniel Kleitman        Sleep and Wakefulness, Chicago, University of Chicago Press, 1939. 1987 reprint

5          William Dement, M.D. PhD.: The
           Promise of Sleep, Dell Publishing,1999.
6          Allan Rechtschaffen and Anthony Kales:
           A Manual of standardization
           Terminology, Techniques and Scoring
           System for Sleep Stages of Human
           Subjects. US Department of Health,
           Education, and Welfare Public Health
           Service, NIH/NIND,   1968
7          Robert Stickgold, PhD.: Sleep, Memory
           and Dreams: Extracting the Meaning of
           our Lives. Plenary Session of APSS 2013.
8          James K. Wyatt: Sleep Onset is
           Associated with Retrograde and
           Anterograde Amnesia.     Sleep
           17(6):502-511. 1994
9          Martin Moore-Ede: Circadian
           Timekeeping in Health and Disease.
           NEJM 309:469-476, 530-536, 1983.
10         Dorsey, C. et al. Core Body Temperature
           and Sleep of Older Female Insomniacs
           Before and After Passive Body Heating.
           SLEEP, Vol 22, No 7, 1999.
11         Consensus Conference Panel, Watson
           NF et al. Recommended Amount of
           Sleep for a Healthy Adult: A Joint
           Consensus Statement of the American
           Academy of Sleep Medicine and Sleep
           Research Society. Journal of Clinical
           Sleep Medicine, Vol. 11, No. 6, 2015.

12      A.A. Borbely: Sleep: circadian rhythm vs. recovery process. In KMLDaA J (ed): Functional States of the Brain: Their Determinants. Amsterdam, Elsevier/North -Holland, 1980, pp151-161.

13      Eun-Ok Im, PhD MPH FAAN et al. Sleep related symptoms of Midlife women with and without type 2 diabetes mellitus.

14      Rogerio A. Lobo. Menopause. Cecil's Textbook of Medicine, 22 edition, pp1533-1539. 2004.

15      S.S. Yen: The biology of Menopause. Journal of Reproductive Medicine, 1977;18-287

16      Anjel Vahratian. NCHS Data Brief No. 286, September 2017. Sleep Duration and Quality Among women Aged 40-59, by Menopausal Status

17      Reddy, S. et al. Gabapentin, Estrogen, and Placebo for Treating Hot Flashes. Obstetrics and Gynecology, Vol. 108, No.1, July 2006.

18      Shams, T. et al. SSRIs for Hot Flashes: A Systematic Review and Meta-Analysis of Randomized Trials. Journal of General Internal Med 29 (1): 204-13.

19      Ong, TH et al. Simplifying STOP-
        BANG: use of a simple questionnaire to
        screen for OSA in an Asian population.
        Sleep Breath. 2010 Dec;14 (4):371-6.

20      Moore, T. et al. Reports of Pathological
        Gambling, Hypersexuality, and
        Compulsive Shopping Associated With
        Dopamine Receptor Agonist Drugs.
        JAMA Intern Med 2014;174(12):1930-
        1933

21      Morin, Charles M. et al. Psychological
        And Behavioral treatment of Insomnia:
        Update Of The Recent Evidence (1998-
        2004) SLEEP, Vol 29, No 11, 2006.

22      Cheng, Philip et al. Journal of Clinical
        Sleep Medicine: Risk of excessive
        sleepiness in sleep restriction therapy and
        cognitive behavioral therapy for
        insomnia: a randomized controlled trial.
        Vol 16.  No 2. Feb 15, 2020.

23      Chen, L et al. Journal of Clinical Sleep
        Medicine: Effects of an Acute Bout of
        Light-Intensity Walking on Sleep in
        Older Women with Sleep Impairment: A
        Randomized Controlled Trial